Essential Oils

Practical Aromatherapy Recipes for Natural Soaps, Shampoo and Body Butter

Table of Contents

Introduction

Essential oils have been used since ancient times as a valuable healing tool. The ancient Egyptians are thought to have been the first people to extract these valuable oils and the Romans and the Greeks used them extensively in order to promote healing and good health, as well as for their beautiful and unique scents.

The use of essential oils is commonly referred to as aromatherapy. They can be used to balance both body and mind, and they can have regenerative and restorative properties that can help you to look and feel amazing.

I personally suffer from sensitive skin, and first started making my own products because I was unable to purchase anything that didn't irritate my skin for less than one hundred dollars. I now make all of my family's cleaning and beauty products, as well as selling my products both online and locally. This book will allow you to recreate some of my favourite beauty products that are not only effective (I've tested them myself!) but that are also devoid of harsh chemicals.

I will teach you how to make your own soaps, body butters and shampoos, how to choose the best oils for use, how to blend them properly and how to ensure that they are safe and effective. I will also show you how to preserve them naturally so that they last longer!

Once you start to experiment with the oils on your own, you will be astonished at the results that you can achieve over a short period of time. Unlike other natural therapies, essential oils start working from the very first application - there is no need to wait six months to see if the treatment is working.

Your skin and hair will look healthier and be stronger.

Best of all, you can customize your beauty treatments to suit you as a person instead of just buying a generic brand intended for thousands of other clients as well. You will be able to perfectly layer your scents - starting with the soap that you use and finishing off with a matching body butter and perfume - all completely natural without the harsh ingredients found in commercial products.

For most of us, the simple truth is that we are becoming increasingly concerned about what goes into the beauty products that we use on a daily basis. If you want a better solution for both you and your loved ones, my belief is that this book will provide it for you.

Say goodbye to unmanageable hair and skin, and put the control back into your own hands.

Chapter 1:

Making Your Own Beauty Products

Why Commercially Produced Beauty Products Just Don't Make the Cut

Just about everyone will recognize the term "aromatherapy" in some form or another. Whether you have ever used essentials oils yourself, or have seen them dotted all over the beauty aisle in a range of different products, you will have had some exposure to these oils even if you weren't aware of it at the time.

You probably *are* aware of the health benefits of using essential oils - like using Tea Tree oil to help fight against colds and flu - but were you aware that the various oils can be used effectively as beauty treatments as well?

Tea Tree oil, for example, is also a great skin treatment and can clear up acne and cuts and scratches. Palmarosa oil is a wonderful addition to a body butter because it helps the skin to regenerate. Sandalwood oil is deeply moisturizing - the list goes on and on.

Even large commercial companies acknowledge that aromatherapy oils have some value and add these oils to their products. This would seem to be a really great idea until you look a little deeper.

First and foremost, the oils are used in such tiny concentrations that they really do not do any good anyway. Secondly, the products that they are in are likely to contain a range of synthetic chemicals and preservatives - none of which are particularly good for your health.

What you need to remember is that commercially produced products are designed with the sole intent of getting you to buy them. What that means is that they are often contain little extras that you really do not need. I will bet, for example, that you always thought that the shampoo had to lather to be effective, didn't you? Well, so does everyone and that is why ingredients are added to help the shampoo lather. In fact, it is when shampoo encounters dirty hair that it less likely to lather meaning that the more the shampoo lathers, the cleaner your hair already is.

Companies want the longest shelf-life that they can get and will add preservatives to keep their product going for longer.

In addition, they add a whole lot of other things to make their product appear to work better and smell better, leaving you with a wholly synthetic product overall. Why on earth would you want to subject yourself to that when there are a lot of better options available?

Modern aromatherapy was "rediscovered" by a Frenchman named Gattefosse. He was working in his family's perfumery lab one day when he burnt his hand quite severely. The only liquid nearby was a vat of Lavender oil and so he immediately put his hand into it.

When he realized that the burn was healing a lot faster than normal and that there was no blistering, he began to become obsessed with the healing benefits of essential oils and started more research into them.

A French woman, Marguerite Maury, developed the principles of conventional aromatherapy that we follow today - she researched effective methods of dilution and application through massage.

In the last couple of decades, there has been a resurgence in interest in natural remedies as we begin to realize that there are very real, negative long term side effects associated with synthetically-manufactured medications and products.

More and more evidence is surfacing that essential oils can be just as effective as more conventional treatments but without the negative side effects.

Why should you use aromatherapy in your beauty products? Well, the fact is that you probably already are to a small extent.

Essential oils are derived from various different parts of the plant - the petals, roots, bark, peel, fruit or resin. You may come in contact with the same essences during the course of your day - take the lemon that you use for your detox drink. It is strongly scented and just through smelling the peel, you are benefiting from the essence of the plant itself.

You are basically giving yourself an aromatherapy treatment quickly and easily so why not go the whole hog and learn a bit more about using essential oils in your beauty routine as well?

Now, obviously the essential oil of a plant is a lot more concentrated than the essence that you get out of just one piece, but the idea is still the same.

Chapter 2:

Important Safety Information

Read This BEFORE You Start With Your Recipes

First and foremost, let us get the safety aspects out of the way. Essential oils are natural but you do have to take some basic precautions in order to be able to use them safely and effectively.

The oils themselves are the distilled, highly concentrated compounds of the plants that they are derived from, in liquid form and this is what makes them so powerful but it is also why we need to be a bit more careful in how we apply them.

The concentrated format of the oils means that they are hundreds or thousands of times more powerful than the compounds found in nature. This makes sense because of the vast amounts of plant matter that need to be processed in order to produce just one small bottle of essential oils. That one bottle of oil contains the healing power of all the hundreds or thousands of petals/ leaves/ roots that went into the making of the oil.

Use the Best Quality That You Can Afford

There are a lot of commercial products on the market that purport to contain essential oils. They probably do but the concentrations of essential oils in bath oils, shampoos, etc. is negligible and not likely to do you any good at all. These products may smell nice but this is not what I mean when I say that you need to incorporate essential oils into your life. You need to find 100% pure essential oils. This may mean going to a specialist store, health store or possibly searching online for the right product. In the end, the extra effort will be well worth it at the end of the day.

There are a range of products in the same aisle as the essential oils in the store. It is important to get the purest grade that you can afford - in fact, it is better to not buy any oils at all than to settle for second-grade, adulterated oils. It is also important to choose a company that has a proven track record and that will not try to pull the wool over your eyes when it comes to the oils that they sell.

The oils should say, "Therapeutic Grade" or "100% Pure". The oil should also list both the common name and the botanical name. Good companies also list how the product was distilled and which region it originally came from.

Where the Oil is Sourced

Believe it or not, there can be a difference in the components in the oils that is region-specific. Lavender that is grown in France, for example, can be very different to that grown in the United States, even if they are the exact same species. The soil the plant is grown in, the local weather conditions and even the way it has been stored all influence the components in the oil that is eventually distilled. These components can even vary in the same field of plants from year to year. That said, don't get too bogged down by this - choose a reputable company to deal with and you can be assured that you do get what you are paying for.

How are the Oils Extracted?

The process by which the oils are extracted is also important. Oils may be extracted through the use of solvents - this is usually the case with resinous oils and oils that would be damaged due to high heat due to distillation - and this is the least expensive means of extraction. The problem is that the cheaper brands of oils are generally going to contain a higher residue of these solvents.

Water or steam distillation is a more common means of extraction for higher quality oils and is used in 90% of cases. Two examples of oils that have to be extracted using solvents are Jasmine and Benzoin oil. They would not survive the distillation process.

Be Careful Of

Words to watch out for are "Blend" or "Fragrance Oil". In the first case, the company should list exactly what oils have been used to bolster the blend. If they are honest about this, you might still be able to use the oil - just check that the oils blended in are also suitable for use on babies and kids.

Blending pure oils with less expensive ones that have similar properties or fragrance is common practice. Rose essential oil is often blended with Geranium essential oil, for example. The reason for this is that Rose absolute is ridiculously expensive to produce and most people would not be able to afford to use the absolute anyway. This need not be an issue, as long as the company does this openly. The problem comes in when you get a less scrupulous company that makes no mention that the oil has been adulterated.

Price is a Fair Indicator of Quality

Price is pretty much your best indication of this sharp practice. These company's usually charge a fair amount less for their oils and may even charge the same price for every oil in the range. If the price seems too good to be true, it probably is. If the prices across the range of oils for one company seem about the same, you should avoid that brand - essential oils should vary in price according to how easily they are distilled, how much plant material is used, and how common the plant is, they should never be all that same price.

Fragrance Oils Should be Banned!

Step away from the Fragrance oils, these should never enter your home. They may smell similar to the oils but they have been synthetically produced and so have no medicinal properties whatsoever. These oils are really a cheap substitute (and here I use the word "substitute" very lightly because they really are completely different from pure essential oils. They are generally made up using cheap solvents and chemicals so I keep them far away from my kids. They should certainly never be applied to the skin - they will definitely irritate the skin and I personally don't think that they should even be inhaled. Who knows what chemicals they use?

Always Pay Attention to Dilution Rules

It is because of this high concentration of compounds that you should dilute the oils before applying them to the skin. And this applies to all essential oils, even Tea Tree oil and Lavender oil. Tea Tree oil and Lavender oil are a lot gentler on the skin and are technically gentle enough to be used neat, but may cause sensitization, especially when used on children and especially when it comes to broken skin.

To be on the safe side, I simply hardly ever use essential oils unless they have been diluted first - whether I am applying them directly to the skin or putting them in the bath water. At best, neat oils might cause irritation, at worst, they might burn the skin.

Many books will say that you can apply neat Tea Tree oil or Lavender oil to scratches, bites, etc. When it comes to babies and toddlers under the age of 6 months, this is definitely not something to take a chance with. The oils are very powerful, even when diluted, so they will still have a strong healing effect even when applied in small quantities like for a shampoo or soap.

Keep Out of the Reach of Little Fingers

I learned this the hard way when my nephew was about two. Like all my kids, he was a real little monkey and managed to clamber up onto the Welsh dresser to get at my bottles of essential oils. It never once occurred to me that he would clamber up. (Though looking back on it now, he was a really clever little kid and got himself into loads of sticky situations.)

He managed to open the Eucalyptus oil (kids learn quickly and a bottle is there to be opened, as far as they are concerned - never be complacent and think that anything is safe from a kid) and slapped drops of it onto his face. He had applied about a quarter bottle before it started to sting. Fortunately I got to him quickly and wiped his face down before it got a chance to burn but his cheeks were quite red and I learned a valuable lesson - keep the oils where the kids cannot possibly get to them. I just count my lucky stars that he didn't get it into his head to drink the oils and that, because of the dropper, they only came out a little at a time. Since that time, I lock all my essential oils away.

Should the same thing happen to you, take a wet facecloth and wipe away the oils - don't forget to wipe any residue off their fingers as well - and then apply plain aqueous cream. This will help to both dilute any oils that were absorbed and soothe the stinging.

If the child gets any oils in the eyes or their mouth, your best bet is to wash the areas with milk first. The essential oils are not soluble in water and so will not be absorbed by it when it comes to the mucous membranes of the mouth or the sensitive cornea of the eye. They are, however, soluble in milk so the milk is the better option to clean out some of the essential oils. Afterwards, you can rinse with tepid water.

If the skin or eyes are burned, get the child to the emergency room as quickly as possible and be sure to tell them what oils the child used.

Taking the Oils Internally

There are people out there that advocate adding the oils to your daily diet. This is irresponsible advice at best and can actually be quite dangerous. The oils can be toxic if taken internally, even in small doses. If you suspect that your child has swallowed even a few milliliters of these oils, try and force them to vomit and get them to the doctor as quickly as possible. As little as 4ml of Eucalyptus oil, for example, can be a lethal dose.

The confusion actually came about because in French aromatherapy there is a place for the internal use of oils. It is a valid form of French aromatherapy. What should be remembered, however, is that this takes place under the supervision of a highly trained and qualified aromatherapist. For the amateur at home, it is too dangerous to take any risks and the potential rewards are simply not worth the risk.

The oils are absorbed through the skin and through inhalation a lot more quickly than would be the case if they had to work their way through your digestive system first.

NOT for Newborns

It is not advisable to start using essential oils on your baby before they are 10 weeks old. This is because their immune systems are still developing and introducing the oils at this stage could cause them to develop allergies. After they are 10 weeks old, you can start introducing the more gentle oils, such as Lavender and Chamomile.

When you do start to introduce the oils, even after the baby is 10 weeks old, you still need to check that there are no adverse reactions to the oils. Doing a patch test on the skin first and waiting for at least 12 hours to see whether or not there are any adverse reactions is really important.

If you are unsure of whether or not the oil is going to irritate the skin or not, rather diffuse a small amount of the oil in the baby's general vicinity. This can be as powerful as applying the oils to the skin, without risking irritating the baby's sensitive skin.

Again, when diffusing the oils for the first few times, watch your baby to see whether or not there are any adverse reactions - if you see signs that they are in distress or battling to breathe, get them away from the area immediately.

The Dosage Must be Right

Your child's age and size need to be taken into consideration when deciding on the appropriate dose. In general, the smaller the child, the lower the dose. Think about it for a second - your child's body is a lot smaller than yours - just as you reduce the strength of shampoo used for them, you need to do the same when it comes to essential oils.

Photo-Toxic Oils

Some oils, particularly citrus oils, are photo-toxic. This is not as bad as it sounds, all it means is that the oils will react to the sun or UV light and that this can sensitize the skin, cause discoloration or a rash. When using these oils, make sure that you will not be exposed to sunlight for at least a couple of hours. For safety sake, I reserve these oils for use in the early evening.

Store Carefully

To get the best benefits from your essential oils, you need to ensure that they are stored away from light at a fairly even, cool temperature. The same applies to the carrier oils that you will be using so it does make good sense to find a space for them in the cupboard under the stairs or in the basement. The bathroom seems like a logical space to keep the oils but, due to the amount of steam and moisture, it really is not.

Wherever you decide to store them, keep them under lock and key, especially if you have curious kids or kids that are able to walk. (Remember the lesson I learned and learn from that.)

After use be sure to close all bottles tightly to avoid the loss of oils through evaporation.

Beware of Rancid Oils

Whilst essential oils are not technically oils, they can go off after a while. Their useful lifespan will depend on the oil itself, the quality of the oil and how well they have been stored. Citrus oils, for example, tend to lose effectiveness much faster than the others and are a lot more sensitive to light and oxidation. You are typically looking at around 6 month to a couple of years. It makes sense for you to really only buy the oils that you need as you find that you need them.

Carrier oils also have a sell-by date, again, around 6 months to a couple of years and, again, depending on the type of oil, the quality of the oil and how well it has been stored. Avoid buying large quantities of carrier oils unless you are sure that you will be able to use them before they turn rancid.

The same can be said of blends. Adding a fixative oil, such as Sandalwood or Cedar Wood, for example, can extend the useful lifespan of a blend of oils and help to stabilize more volatile oils but even this will only go so far.

With both essential oils and carrier oils, changes in smell, color and texture are indicative that the oil is past its expiry date and should be thrown out. Using rancid oils will end up being a waste of time at best and can cause irritation or sensitization at best so don't take a chance - if in doubt, throw it out.

Special Circumstances

Not all oils are suitable for everyone so it is advisable, if you have a medical condition, or are pregnant, to get the advice of a qualified aromatherapist before using any of the remedies in this book or using any essential oils at all. Rosemary oil, for example, can raise the blood pressure and can induce uterine contractions causing a miscarriage. Whilst most oils are safe, it is better to be safe than sorry - check with a professional first.

Keep it Simple

You might be keen to try and blend several oils together to get the benefits of all of them. As long as the oils all blend together well, this will not be an issue. If they are not compatible with one another, they will actually work against one another making the blend ineffective. You will normally be able to tell if a blend is bad by the way it smells - when the wrong oils are mixed together the blend will normally smell bland at best and awful at worst.

Start out learning about what works by using the recipes in this book - you can always experiment later on down the line. When you do start to make your own blends, it is best to blend no more than two or three oils initially.

The other problem when your recipes become too complicated is that it is then much harder to determine which oil is at fault if irritation or an allergic reaction does take place. To start off with, do a small patch test with the oil you want to use mixed into some carrier oil. If no reactions occur, you can then add it to your soaps, shampoos, etc.

I would also advise investing in a directory of essential oils if this field really interests you so that you can see what oils are good for medicinal uses as well.

Keep a Record

I always keep a record of every new blend that I have made. I note down what I like about the blend and what I don't like. I also note what my reactions are and what actual effect the oils are having.

I have learned over the years that it is better to write down your recipes as you are making them. It only takes a few seconds extra but can save you hours of extra effort in the long-term. I still have my original notebook that I started out with years ago - it is now, however, looking a bit worse for wear but I do still refer to it often, especially when it comes to beauty products.

The shampoos, etc. make great gifts but you need to be able to remember what you put into them because, most of the time, you will find that you will be asked for refills. There really is nothing as frustrating as finding the perfect body butter blend and forgetting what you had put into it.

Getting Blending Right

When trying a new blend, us no more than 10ml-20ml of your chosen carrier oil. That way, you won't worry about wasting ingredients. This is important because blending is largely a matter of personal taste.

Choose two to three essential oils and add them in one drop at a time, smelling the blend after each addition. This may seem painstaking at first but once you have the blend right, it will be worth it.

If one of the oils that you are using seems to be overpowering the others, add more of the lighter oils to compensate. Sandalwood, for example, is a very fragrant oil. When mixing it in a blend, I will often use it as a base and use only one part Sandalwood for every two parts of the other oils.

Do take notes and watch the concentration of the oils - add more carrier oil as needed, it won't affect the scent much at all.

Hit the Right Notes

Of course, getting the blend right means that it will smell a whole lot better. The perfume industry has this down to a fine art and you can take a note or two from their book.

A cologne or perfume hardly ever smells exactly the same on two different people because of different body chemistry. The scent also smells different over time once applied. At first, you get the heady blend of aroma, this settles down to a fuller aroma over time and finally the scent settles to its base notes.

The secret to a good blend is to blend a more volatile oil, such as Jasmine, with an oils that has a little more staying power, such as Neroli and then to finally add an oil that acts as a fixative for both, like Sandalwood. In this case, Jasmine is the top note, the fragrance that is initially smelt and quickly dissipates. Neroli is the scent that forms the bulk of the blend or the middle note and Sandalwood is the lingering fragrance or base note.

Label Everything

I also suggest labelling the jars - all you need to do is to write which oils you used and the number of drops of each oil. If you want, you can assign a number to the blend in the book or a special name for each blend and cross reference it to the book when you need to but I find that it is usually just quicker to write out the label. At the very least, record what the blend is for on the label.

Cover the label with an adhesive plastic or cello tape so that it is completely protected from cream/ oil spills. (If you don't, the label may become unreadable over time)

Don't skip this step, it really doesn't take long and you will kick yourself for not doing it when faced with a half-full bottle of shampoos and buddy butters that you cannot identify - you will not always be able to identify the blend through scent alone. I have thrown out many a half-filled bottle of oils because I couldn't remember what was in them and didn't want to risk using the wrong oils.

Patch Tests

When trying out a new product, always do a patch test on your skin first. If it irritates your skin, you need to dilute the blend further and try again. Children's skin is bound to be more sensitive than yours so if it is irritating to your skin, it is bound to be worse for your child. When you are happy that the blend is non-irritant, apply the precautions when applying the blend to your child. Do a patch test and wait at least 6-12 hours to see whether the skin reacts badly.

Do this whenever you try a completely new oil or a new blend. Also do it when you get in a new batch of oils, even if they have been fine previously and when you have made any batch of oils from scratch. It pays to also be careful with oils/blends that have been sitting at the back of the cupboard for a while - they might have gone off since you last used them.

Glass is Better

Glass is always better to use and quite easy to lay hands on. I suggest using a shallow jar with a wide mouth for the body butters because they are not as viscous as lotions and a bottle with a narrow neck for the shampoos so that you can more easily control the flow out of the bottle.

Plastic will do in a pinch but if you are really serious about reducing the amount of chemicals in your life, glass is the safer choice. It is better for you because it is not degrade and it is better for the environment because it is recyclable.

You can also recycle old glass jars as long as you ensure that they are washed out in warm soapy water and that no hint of the previous content remains. Food smells in the jar could contaminate your body butters or shampoos and ruin the smell.

If you are planning on adding organic matter to your creams, you must ensure that you do sterilize the bottles before use to lessen the chance of bacterial growth.

It is important to choose glass bottles that do close well to improve the shelf-life and scent of your products.

More is not Necessarily Better

Many of us make the mistake of thinking that if a little of something will work, a lot of it will work far better. When it comes to making your own beauty products, this is not the case at all.

The higher the concentration of oils in the products, the greater the chances that irritation will develop or a tolerance will build. Let's say that you make a soap to clear up acne, for example, and you decide to add the highest allowable quantity of oils to make the soap extra strong. It may end up being too strong or, worse still, the skin may get used to the oils used and develop a tolerance for that particular soap. Then what do you do? You cannot increase the dosage again and will need to start from scratch.

Always start with the lowest possible concentration and, if you are finding that this does not work, then start increasing it slowly. With shampoos and body butters, this simply means adding in some extra drops of the essential oils. Soaps are a little more tricky but nothing stops you from re-batching the soaps in order to be able to add in more of the essential oils.

Chapter 3: How to Choose What Oils to Use

Why Smell Should Be a Secondary Consideration

We all like our beauty products to smell nice but is smell is your only consideration when choosing the essential oils to use, then it may pay you to simply stick to commercial products.

The way the product smells is important but this is secondary to choosing oils with the right properties. For example, if you have dry hair, Rosemary oil is not the best oil as it is better suited to dry hair conditions.

When choosing an oil you also need to consider how easy it is to blend, how it will be applied, when it will be applied and whether or not you like the smell.

Oils that are potentially irritating for the skin, like Cinnamon, for example, should not be used in a body butter.

Then, of course, you need to consider how many oils you will blend into your products. You need to ensure that each oil not only has the right benefits but also that it will blend in with all the other oils as well.

The last consideration is whether or not you like the smell - if you do not, are you going to use the product created? If you are creating a product for others, consider what they would like as well.

Looking for Oils that Play Well With Others

Essential oils are very potent and blending synergistic oils can make them even more so. You can create a much more effective beauty treatment by blending two or more oils together.

Some oils, such as Lavender oil, blend easily with others. Others, such as Tea Tree oil, do not blend that well with many other oils. If you need to choose between two oils to keep in your kit, I would advise choosing the oil that is easier to blend. This will allow you to make a much wider variety of products in future.

The Products the Oils Will Be Used to Create

When it comes to beauty products, this is going to mean either in a cream base, as a shampoo or hair treatment or in a soap. You will need to do a bit of homework beforehand to make sure that the essential oil in question will be the correct one for this type of application. A resinous oil, like Vertiver, for example, may be perfect to blend in a soap but not such a great addition to a shampoo. If you want to use it as a hair treatment, a hot oil treatment could be the better option for you.

What Time of Day Will You Be Using the Products?

When you are going to apply the oils is also important. You need to remember that the oils act not only on the physical body but also on the mind. Using Rosemary oil, for example, in a shampoo for greasy hair can be very helpful - but not if you are going to apply it in the hours leading up to bedtime. Rosemary oil is a powerful mental stimulant and you are likely to have trouble sleeping. Using it in the morning, on the other hand, can set you up for the whole day.

Citrus oils, as another example, can cause your skin to become more photo-sensitive so it is not a good idea to apply these before going out into the sun. These oils are best reserved for use in soaps and shampoos unless you only apply the body butter at night.

Whether or Not you Like the Smell

My mother used to tell me that the worse I thought my medicine tasted, the better it actually was for me. In aromatherapy, the opposite is true.

Whilst the properties of the oil are not affected by whether or not you like its smell, its overall efficacy is. It's simple - the better you like the smell, the better your mind will respond to it.

I, for example, do not like the smell of lavender essential oil. Despite the fact that it is one of the most soothing oils, if I put a few drops on my pillow, I quickly get annoyed with the smell and have to swap the pillow out. Therefore it would really be a stretch for me to use heavily scented Lavender Body Butter. Personally I prefer the soothing scent of Sandalwood.

Your own preferences will be different so I advise you to play around with the different groups of scents to narrow down the scents that you like best. Perhaps you prefer the fresh smell of citrus oils, or perhaps you prefer the scent of the floral oils. Your personal preferences are worth determining if you are going to be making your own beauty products.

The Top Oils for Use in Bath and Beauty Products

Basil Oil: Basil is one of those oils that is not absolutely essential but it is a good oil to have on hand if you have teens that need to study for exams or if you yourself need to study or focus. It doesn't seem to really fit with beauty products but mixing it with Bergamot and Lime and you get a surprisingly fresh fragrance. Mixing it with Citronella will mean that insects will give you a wide berth. It is not safe to use during pregnancy and may irritate the skin so it should not be used in a soap. It can be used in your body butter if very heavily diluted. It can also be added to shampoo to get similar benefits to the diffused oil. It is a good remedy for respiratory tract infections, colds, the flu and other infectious illnesses and it can clear out a brain fog quite fast. It is a good treatment for stress, anxiety, depression and fatigue. Blended in low concentrations it is good for treating stomach upsets and menstrual cramping. It can help to relieve the pain associated with gout and also sore muscles and joints.

Benzoin: You may find that Benzoin is one of those oils that is a little more difficult to find a spot for in a blend but then again, even used on its own, its permeating vanilla scent is often enough to lift the spirits. It can help ease a tight chest and is very valuable in the treatment of depression and stress. Blend equal parts Benzoin oil, Rose oil and Jasmine oil for a truly heavenly blend that smells wonderful and that will lift your spirits in no time flat. This is a very sluggish liquid as it is derived from a resin and so I find that it is better used in a soap. A drop or so is all that is needed - it has a very rich aroma. Mixed with 2 drops each of Cedar Wood oil and Neroli oil in a diffuser and you have the perfect blend to use when feeling overworked and under pressure.

Bergamot Oil: Bergamot is quite a useful oil to have - it has strong anti-bacterial properties and is also an effective fungus fighter. It is good for treating vaginal discharge, cystitis, acne, boils, cold sores, eczema, insect repellent and insect bites, oily complexion, psoriasis, scabies, spots, varicose ulcers, wounds. It is a good oil to use to counter depression and to also combat sleeplessness caused by depression. It will work in a soap, shampoo or body butter. It can cause photo-sensitivity so do take care when using it in sunlight.

Carrot Seed Oil: This is one of the best skin healers and rejuvenators. It helps to improve skin turnover and helps to reduce the appearance of stretch marks and scars. Mixed with equal quantities of Palmarosa oil into a body butter, this is perfect for use after baby is born to help the skin recover. It can help to treat a dry, itchy scalp if incorporated into a shampoo.

Chamomile Oil: Chamomile oil is another one of those must-have oils. It does have a very sweet smell so you will either love it or be indifferent to it but it is also another of the gentle oils that can be used on babies over the age of 10 weeks. It is the oil that has the strongest analgesic properties and it blends very well with Lavender to create a potent headache treatment. Just use as a cold compress applied to the back of the neck and rub a few drops of the blend into each temple.

If your baby is teething or if you have a tooth ache, Chamomile is very effective at relieving that throbbing pain. Apply a blend of Chamomile and Lavender to the outside of the mouth where the trouble is. A couple of drops massaged into the outside of the ear can help to soothe earache. It will also help to reduce anxiety and stress - it is ideal to soothe a toddler who is battling with teething pains and can effectively put a stop to a temper tantrums.

It can relieve aching muscles and joints - it is a strong anti-inflammatory. It is also a very effective anti-spasmodic as a topical treatment - use for menstrual cramping or stomach troubles. It can help to soothe allergic skin reactions and eczema. It helps to soothe dry, troubled skin - mix with Lavender and Sandalwood for a wonderful treatment for skin that is suffering from exposure.

Eucalyptus Oil: Eucalyptus should definitely be a part of your kit if you are an athlete or avid sportsperson - it is really great for soothing stiff and sore muscles. It is also essential if you have young kids or if you or anyone in your family is prone to getting respiratory tract infections. Eucalyptus oil has quite a strong scent and has strong anti-bacterial and anti-viral properties. It is wonderful for unblocking a stuffy nose and relieving the symptoms and aches of cold and the flu. It is also great for getting rid of a sinus headache. Rub a blend of Eucalyptus and Lavender oil into the feet at night to help the body fight infection and to help break a fever. Used in a skin care blend, very diluted, it can also help to fight infections of the skin. Diffuse it when sitting outside on the patio on the insects will leave you alone. If you are battling with cellulite, a daily massage with a Eucalyptus blend will help detoxify and smooth skin and also boost circulation.

Frankincense Oil: If you have troubled skin, this is the ideal oil to add to your soap - it helps fight the bacteria and inflammation of acne and pimples and it helps to protect your skin cells from damage. It also encourages the growth of new cells and can be very effective at reducing wrinkles, firming up skin and lightening scars. It is a soother for dry and chapped skin as well.

Geranium Oil: As far as the skin is concerned, this is one of the most useful oils. It helps to balance the production of sebum and so is good in a soap for treating troubled skin. It is deeply nourishing and helps to prevent dry, tight skin and also reduces the formation of wrinkles. It helps to lighten scars and stretchmarks. It is a good addition to a body butter if you bruise easily or if you have poor circulation or varicose veins. It is anti-fungal, anti-bacterial and anti-inflammatory. It can soothe contact dermatitis, eczema and itchy rashes and can help to reduce the appearance of broken capillaries on the face. This is your skin's best friend. For your hair, it can help to balance out sebum production on the scalp as well and makes a great addition to a dry shampoo if you have greasy hair.

Jasmine Oil: Jasmine absolute is rather expensive and, to be honest, out of most people's price ranges. That is not to say that you can never use it - Jasmine blends are available on the market and some of these are actually pretty good. If you want to add Jasmine oil, stick to only a well-known, quality brand. You will pay extra but this is one of the most useful oils when it comes to creating feeling of content and in beating back depression. Jasmine oil also has wonderful curative properties for the skin and will blend with almost all other essential oils. It can also help ease a hoarse throat. Jasmine is a floral note and is quite penetrating so start with lower concentrations. If you want to make floral perfumes or perfumes with a hint of the Orient, Jasmine is an oil that you must get. It helps to round off the more severe notes and to harmonize the blend overall.

Lavender Oil: If Mother Nature was a snake oil salesman, this would be her tonic to cure everything. The difference being that in the case of Lavender oil and your skin, this is no idle boast. One of the few oils that can be applied neat, Lavender oil can find a place in body butters, shampoos and soaps to promote skin regeneration and to help improve skin turnover. It is deeply nourishing and so ideal for very dry skin or hair. It can also help to balance sebum production and so can also be used on greasy hair. In fact, it will work wonders on any skin and hair type.

Lemon Oil: Lemon oil is a great natural astringent and has very strong anti-bacterial properties. It is great to get troubled, oily skin under control and will help to refine the pores. As such, it works well in a soap. There is on caveat though, it should never be used on the skin just before going out into the sun as it is highly photo-sensitive. If you do want to venture out after using it, be sure to wear sunscreen. For hair, it is best for greasy to normal hair types. If you like, you can also take advantage of the photo-sensitive properties to lighter your hair by washing your hair with a Lemon oil shampoo and sitting in the sun until your hair is dry.

Myrrh Oil: Myrrh oil is a deeply nourishing oil that has great benefits for very dry or mature skin and hair. It helps to reduce the damage caused by exposure to the sun, helps to relieve skin conditions such as eczema and rashes and can help to tone and tighten the skin, help the skin to regain elasticity and also reduce the look of wrinkles and other fine lines.

Neroli Oil: Neroli Water, made from the water left over in the process of extracting the oils has been used for centuries as a beauty treatment. The legend has it that Elizabeth, Queen of Hungary in the 1300's used it as a daily beauty treatment and so even managed to snag a husband many years her junior because she still looked so beautiful. Neroli oil itself is really good for all skin tones but works especially well for sensitive and dry skins. It does have oil balancing properties and will smooth out wrinkles and help to restore the skin's elasticity. It is also a really excellent treatment for the prevention of stretch marks and reducing their appearance. It blends well with Geranium, Sandalwood and Palmarosa oil for use in a body butter to combat eczema and extremely dry skin conditions.

Patchouli Oil: Patchouli works well when it comes to mature skin. It encourages skin turnover and reduces the appearance of wrinkles and fine lines. It can combat infections of the skin and help to sooth inflammatory skin conditions. It works best when used on normal to dry hair.

Peppermint: I'm pretty sure that you have heard about the digestion soothing effects of Peppermint tea. The essential oil is equally as useful but also has a few uses that you may not have known about. Peppermint's regulating effects on the digestive system make it a truly useful herb and one that does deserve a place in the top ten. It can help to ease dyspepsia, indigestion, colic and flatulence. It also has strong anti-spasmodic properties making it a valuable addition to a post-workout blend. In addition, is aids circulation, warms muscles and soothes aches in muscles and joints. I do avoid using the oil on my face and do only use it at a maximum of 1% dilution as it may cause irritation to the skin.

I find that the oil is especially useful in the treatment of head colds - there is nothing better to clear up a nasty sinus infection than a blend of Peppermint, Eucalyptus and Lavender oils. I use this oil a lot when I need to focus - it is a very stimulating oil and clears out foggy thinking very fast. It should not be used near to bedtime as it can keep you awake. It can also interfere with the efficacy of homeopathic treatments and should never be used by pregnant women.

Rose Oil: This is another of Mother Nature's greatest hits. It is especially for dry or mature skin. It helps to heal the skin and reduces the signs of aging, it tones and refines the skin and can reduce inflammation and the redness associated with broken capillaries. It makes a great scent addition to a shampoo and can help to treat a dry scalp and dandruff.

Rosemary: Rosemary is another of those scents that you will either love or hate. It is quite a strong scent and can be overpowering in a blend so again, use 2 drops of your other oils with every 1 drop of Rosemary oil. This is one oil that is very good for oily skin and is useful in the treatment of acne. It is too harsh for dry or sensitive skin though. It is a great oil to help stimulate hair growth - rub a blend of Rosemary and Lavender into the scalp just about half an hour before washing your hair to help promote hair growth and a healthy scalp (Preferably not within 2-3 hours of bedtime).

It is a very effective stimulant for the circulatory system and warms muscles. It has analgesic properties so is particularly good for those suffering from muscle stiffness and soreness, especially when this is due to overwork. It can also be valuable in relieving arthritic and rheumatic pain.

Rosemary oil is a good tonic for the liver and gallbladder so rub over the abdomen after over-indulging. Rosemary oil is very effective at treating disorders of the respiratory system such as sinusitis and bronchitis. Blend with eucalyptus to ease coughing and wheezing. Rosemary is also very useful in the treatment of headaches, especially if these are brought on by stress and tension. Apply as a cool compress to the back of the neck. In ancient times, Roman soldiers would tuck a sprig of Rosemary behind their ears to help them focus their attention. This tactic is just as effective when using Rosemary oil. When I really need to focus on writing or studying, I blend together Rosemary oil and Lime oil and massage it into my scalp. I find that this helps me to focus for longer periods of time and let's me work longer and harder, with less chance of fatigue setting in.

Sandalwood: Sandalwood oil is one of the more expensive oils but a little really goes a long way. It is a superb fixative oil and blends well with many different oils. I have to admit that this is one of my favorite oils. I also find that I use it a lot. If the cost is too much for you, Cedar Wood oil has similar properties but is more affordable. Sandalwood is particularly important if you have mature, dry skin.

Mixed into a blend of Neroli, Palmrosa and Lavender, it is a potent anti-wrinkle treatment to use at night. It is a great sinus cleanser and will help alleviate dry coughs and the symptoms of colds and the flu. Where it really shines though is in its ability to help you to relax and relieve nervous tension, especially when these are a result of a fear of change. As a fixative, there is no oil to match it. I once made a batch of aqueous cream, using Sandalwood as the fixative and no preservatives. The bottle rolled under a bookcase and I forgot about it. A couple of years later, we moved house and the bottle was found. The blend still smelled as good as it had on the day it was blended.

Sweet Marjoram: This is not an oil that is commonly recommended in popular magazines, etc. and I think that this is such a pity. Whilst this is not an oil that I would use in perfumery because it has a strong scent, I do find that its other qualities more than make up for this. I find that it is particularly useful for relieving tired and sore muscles and joints, especially if blended with a little Lavender oil. It warms the muscles and is very soothing overall. If you battle with circulatory problems or high blood pressure, this is one oil that should be on your shopping list - it can help reduce bruising, regulate blood pressure and also prevent chilblains. It has strong anti-bacterial and anti-viral properties making it useful in the treatment of colds and the flu. Mixed with Chamomile and Lavender oils, it makes a soothing rub for a tight chest and wracking cough. It has anti-spasmodic properties and can be used in a warm compress to help alleviate menstrual cramps and pain. It helps to regulate the menstrual cycle, particularly when blended with Clary Sage. For me personally, it is its calming effect that is most helpful. If I find that I am feeling panicky or over-anxious, Sweet Marjoram blended with either Lime or Chamomile always helps me put things back into perspective. Mixed with Lavender and Chamomile, this makes a really effective treatment for headaches and migraines - massage into the temple or use as a cool compress over the forehead and at the back of the neck

Tea Tree Oil: Most people by now have heard about Tea Tree oil. It is the only other oil that can be place neat on the skin and is excellent for spot treating breakouts. It helps to get sebum production under control and so can help troubled skin. It is useful for those with oily hair as well.

Ylang Ylang Oil: This is a richly scented, exotic oil and makes a great addition to soaps and body butters to really take the fragrance factor up a couple of notches. For skin it helps to regulate sebum product and reduces the frequency and severity of breakouts. It can help to balance an oily scalp. It is a great skin regenerator and will improve the overall elasticity and resilience of skin.

Chapter 4:
Creating Your Own Natural Soaps

A Basic Introduction To Natural Soap Crafting

When it comes to basic soap crafting, you might be surprised to learn how simple it can be. There is not even a whole lot of special equipment needed and most of what you need will be able to come from your kitchen. Most of the rest you can pick up inexpensively at a second-hand store.

That said, once you have started using a set of bowls, etc. for soap crafting, you should not use them for preparing food in again. There are two reasons for this - first off, the soap flavor will remain in the food and, secondly, the lye used to make the soaps is highly toxic if ingested in its active form.

It really is not going to be all that difficult to keep a separate set of equipment that you use just for your soaps. Any containers that you use to mix the lye water in need to be very clearly marked so that no one else uses them. They should also be kept out of the reach of kids and pets.

As regards the moulds for your soaps, you can get away with just about anything, as long as you can maneuver the soap out of it. A clean, empty milk carton, foil-lined with with the top cut off makes a perfect mould. The mould should be sturdy but flexible. Steer clear of metal moulds, glass moulds or moulds that are too inflexible. You should also stick to simpler moulds - cold process soap making produces soap that is quite thick and this means that it may not pick up the intricate designs.

If you do not want to make soap from scratch, you can buy a nice castile soap and re-batch it to add in the ingredients that you like. This will involve grating the soap and combining with equal quantities of water. This should be placed on the stove over a double boiler to allow it to heat slowly. Stir gently occasionally and remove from the heat when it is properly combined. Add in whatever ingredients you like and pour into the moulds.

One could fill many books when it comes to how to make your own soap from scratch so I will go through the cliff notes version. There are two basic options - cold-process and hot-process. In the former, the heat required is provided by the heat produced when the lye reacts with the water. For hot-process soap making, you must cook the soap itself.

This book will deal with the cold-process soap making as it produces superior results and has less guesswork involved. The disadvantage, however, is that you need to set the soaps aside to cure for around 6 - 8 weeks before you are able to use them. Another minus is that delicate ingredients can be destroyed during this soap making process.

That is simply remedied, however by making up a plain batch and leaving this to cure. Once that is done, it is quite a simple matter to re-batch the soap - the same way you would if you were using bought castile soap and to add the delicate ingredients at that stage rather.

Hot-processing means that you can use your soap straight away but the soap produced is inferior and you need to carefully watch your soap or risk it burning.

In either event, you will need a dedicated lye container. Because of the acidity of the lye when it mixes with water, it is a good idea to use a glass measuring jug.

You must also be careful when choosing your mixing bowls. If you must have a metal bowl, make sure that it is made from stainless steel. Other metals can react with the lye with disastrous consequences. You bowls should have a pouring lip if possible to make it easier to decant your soap.

Personally, I find that it is better to use glass mixing bowls as I can, when I need to, I just place them in the microwave or over a double boiler so that I can heat the oils in them.

For a mixing spoon, stick to silicone or stainless steel - wood can do in a pinch but the acid will degrade the wood so it is not a long-term solution.

An accurate scale is essential - you have to work with exact quantities. Rubber gloves help to protect your hands and safety glasses should also be brought to bear. I do recommend picking up a handheld blender to mix the soap with to bring it to trace. You can do this by hand but this can take hours. Using the blender takes minutes. I also suggest getting a little coffee grinder, especially if you intend to use bits of organic matter like dried lavender, etc. The particles look pretty in the soap but if they are too big they will make a mess of the bath or shower or even clog the drain.

Whisks in a range of sizes can help to create fun effects. For example, if you beat a soap until it becomes frothy, it will be able to float.

You can make do with a single thermometer but it is far better to use two - the lye solution and the fat need to be at around about the same temperature when you mix them up and so two thermometers are a good idea.

You will need to be able to lay your soap out, preferably slightly raised off the table so that air can circulate around it. I have found that a stainless steel dish-rack or a cutlery drawn both work well for smaller quantities. You can also make your own racks quite easily by making a frame and stapling plastic mesh that the soap can rest on to it. If you like, you can screw in four mini-legs so that the tray is raised off the ground.

Make more racks as needed and ensure the legs are long enough so that you can balance them one on top of the other.

Actually making soap is quite easy. In the early days, all that soap was was a bit of tallow mixed into wood ash and water. There are a good deal more options now but the basic idea is still the same - Fat + Lye = Soap.

You can change things up by using different oils and additives.

In the next chapter, we will go through the basics of what oils and quantities to use to enable you to make the perfect bar of soap.

Chapter 5:

Natural Soaps - Your Recipe Guide

Creating Your Own Recipes From Scratch

This guide will teach you how to set up your own recipes from scratch, going through the quantities required, etc.

Fats

Don't get too carried away when it comes to using all the fats out there. Start off small - my personal favorites are tallow and olive oil. You can also add canola oil, palm oil and coconut oil if you life. I am not fond of coconut oil because I find that it can be drying on the skin and that it might cause rashes when used over an extended period of time. I find that olive oil makes a very firm bar of soap that lasts a long time and is very nourishing. Tallow, for me, makes the nicest lather and has the best feel of all the oils.

Tallow

This is not suitable if you are a vegetarian because it basically is suet that has been boiled to allow the pure fat to rise to the surface and any remaining meat debris to drop to the bottom of the pot. Wherever possible, buy the tallow rather than making your own - it is an unpleasant process and smells bad.

That said, I would render the suet myself if I had to because I really like the feel of this soap - it feels rich and creamy and takes on scents well. It is not going to last as long as a bar made from pure vegetable fat but will trace a lot faster.

You can quite easily make a bar of soap just out of tallow and lye if you want to.

Vegetable Oils

Olive Oil (SAP 0.134)

Olive oil is my favorite when it comes to vegetable oils. tracing time tends to be longer but this is not as much of an issue when you use a hand-held blender to combine the ingredients. It is very mild and very useful in the treatment of bad skin. You can if you like, make a bar of soap out of olive oil and lye. Here it is not vital to look for extra virgin olive oil, even the less refined olive oils will work well. The primary difference being that the less refined olive oil will leave a tinge of green in the soap itself. This though, can also be quite pretty.

Coconut Oil (SAP 0.178)

Coconut oil is not a good oil to use on its own. It is more suited for people with normal/ combination skins. If these are you skin types, coconut oil can make a really good cleanser and possesses anti-bacterial properties as well. It must not, however, make up more than 25% of the fats used for the soap overall or the bar can become brittle.

Canola Oil (SAP 0.132)

If you are working on a tight budget that allow you to use 100% olive oil, this is a fair substitute. Do not, however, use sunflower oil as canola is not that much more expensive and produces a superior bar of soap. The canola will help to lighten the rest of your soap and makes a good lather. You can use up to 35% canola in your fats.

Palm Oil (SAP 0.178)

Palm oil is used extensively in the beauty industry and soap made with it will later well and hold up well. Here you must be careful to stick to a maximum of 15% of the fats or the bar will be very brittle.

Scenting Your Soaps

This is the really fun part when it comes to making soaps - deciding what ingredients to add in. Using 100% pure essential oils will help to ensure that your soaps are effective and that they smell wonderful.

You can use most essential oils for soap making but do need to take note of the possibility that the oils may irritate the skin. It is a bad idea to add Cinnamon oil or Clove oil to a soap because they will both irritate the skin.

If you want to use citrus oils, you can only add them to re-batched soaps. They do not stand up to the soap making process at all well.

Some people are tempted to use fragrance oils, thinking they can save money. Unless these are cosmetic grade oils, don't even consider it. To be honest, the difference in cost between cosmetic grade fragrance oils and essential oils is not really significant enough to warrant swapping for the fragrance oils. Fragrance oils also have no curative benefits and are 100% man-made.

You are looking at somewhere around ½ an ounce to a full ounce of essential oil for every pound of soap made. The amount used will depend on how strong the scent of the oil is and how heavily scented you want the bar to be. Rosemary oil or Tea tree oil, for example have a much stronger scent than Chamomile oil. For the first two oils, ½ an ounce would be plenty. For the Chamomile, you would need to use more oil. Just remember that these are basic guidelines - you need to try them and out and adjust the scent as necessary.

Colorants

I do not believe that one should be using colorants in a natural soap because I believe that the properties of the soap are more important. Many people use mica to color their soaps but considering that there may be heavy metals in them, I don't think that it is worth the risk.

I certainly wouldn't bother going out and buying soap colorants specially. If you want to, add in some coffee grounds or cocoa powder to give the soap a bit of color. Beet and turmeric will also look pretty but considering that the pigments can stain your linen, I do not think that it is worthwhile.

I did have a friend once who used food coloring and that really did not work out well at all.

Additional Ingredients

This is where you can really make your soaps a lot better looking, without resorting to fake colors. Additional ingredients can up the therapeutic value of your soap as well.

Used coffee grounds and ground up oatmeal are excellent exfoliants, for example. The coffee grounds will not only color the soap but also fragrance it as well.

Finely ground pumice can also add an extra element to your soaps, especially where you need a tougher exfoliator.

Finely ground, dried herbs and seeds can be used to create interest as far as the herbs are concerned.

As always, think of safety first when adding additives. The additives should not scratch the skin or cause injury. (Glitter, for example, if it gets in the eye can be quite painful). Also consider whether or not the additives will be able to fit down the plughole without causing a blockage.

Generally speaking, I find that additives are a good way to tell one lot of soap from the next. Perhaps if you are making a few different batches you could add a different additive to each so that you can tell, at a glance, which is which.

Safety and Soap Crafting

Safety when crafting soap should be a priority. Working with lye can be dangerous if you are not careful. Lye or freshly made soap that is spilled on the skin will cause quite painful burns – that is why you should always wear gloves.

The fumes can be noxious so make sure that the area that you are working in is well-ventilated. Safety goggles are a must for protecting your eyes when using lye – if the mixture splashes up into your eyes, it can cause a lot of damage.

You should never put lye into an aluminium container as they react together to form hydrogen gas and this is flammable.

When making your lye solution, always measure out the water first and add the lye to that, rather than the other way round or you could risk the whole mixture exploding.

When adding the lye mixture to your fats, it is important to pour slowly over the back of your spoon so that the mixture does not splash out onto you.

If you have small kids or pets, it is better to keep them out of your work area while making soap – accidents can happen so quickly if you turn your back.

Be careful with the soap mixture – it will be hot at first and the mixture itself will still contain active lye so it can burn the skin if it comes into contact with it. Use gloves when removing the soap from the moulds and don't risk using cold-processed soap before it has fully cured.

Trouble Shooting Your Soaps

Fragrances especially can have a bad reaction with the soap. Here is how to deal with this:

Curdling

Curdling is not necessarily a situation that you cannot recover from. You might still be able to salvage the soap if you whisk or blend well. It should reincorporate itself but, if not, you can try the technique at the end of this chapter.

The Soap Separates

This could be when you have not mixed the mixture properly – it is normally more of a problem when hand-mixing the soap; you have not got the lye calculation correct, the fragrance oil has had a bad effect or there is something wrong with the ingredients that you used.

Again, try stirring the mix to incorporate it. (A hand-held blender works best here.) If that does not work, you can try the method at the end of this chapter.

The Soap Does Not Trace

This is generally a problem when you are mixing by hand – tracing can take hours when mixing by hand. It could also be a problem with one of the ingredients – fragrance oils can prevent tracing or speed it up. The solution is to continue to try and get it to trace. If this doesn't work, try the process at the end of the chapter.

The Soap Seizes

If your soap becomes a hard, lumpy mess, it is most likely due to the addition of a fragrance oil. The only thing that you can do is to try the process at the end of the chapter.

Trying To Salvage Soap

You can try this process to salvage your soap – it should be noted, however, that some batches cannot be saved and that this process does take a bit more effort.

Put on all your safety gear again and pour the ruined batch into a heavy-based pot – stainless steel is your only option here. Your mixture should occupy less than half of the space in the pot.

Using a low-medium heat, warm the soap, stirring often until it becomes like a jelly.

Pour into moulds and leave for few days to harden and then cure as normal.

If this method doesn't work, you will have to throw the batch out. Set it aside to harden and cool completely – this could be a couple of days. Wrap well in bin bags – at least three or four and then throw into the garbage.

A Simple Soap Recipe

Start off with this simple base in order to learn how to get the process going and to get the techniques right. At this point, we are not going to bother with fragrance or color. Get the basic technique right and you can always re-batch this soap later to add fragrance or additives that you like.

In this recipe, the mould is a 1 quart milk or juice container – any container that is waxed. This allows you to experiment before buying too much in the way of specialized equipment. Just be sure to rinse the container really well and let it dry thoroughly before use. Cut off one side rather than the top or bottom as this makes for a more stable container.

You be able to slice it into about 8 decently-sized bars of soap.

3 ounces of Lye

7.26 ounces of water – distilled is best but not essential

4 ounces each of palm and coconut oil

14 ounces of olive oil

Start with the Lye Water. Don your safety goggles and gloves and then set your heat-proof container on the scale, empty. Reset the scale to zero and then add your water until you get the right weight. Set the container that you will be using to measure out the lye on the scale, empty and zero the scale. Weigh the amount of lye that you need.

Now slowly add the lye crystals to the water, stirring slowly and continuously. Try to stand back a little so that you don't breathe in the fumes. Set the water aside. It will be ready to use when it has gone clear again.

Melt the palm oil thoroughly and stir to combine. This is essential when using palm oil. Weigh what you need in a bowl that is big enough to contain all the oils and the lye solution. Melt the coconut oil and add it to the palm oil, stirring continuously. Finally add the olive oil and stir until all the oils are combined.

The lye water and oils should be around the same temperature when combined so set up your thermometers and wait until both mixtures are 120 degrees F.

When both mixtures are roughly the same temperature, add the lye water to the fats slowly – never add the fats to the lye water – pouring over your spoon so that there are no splashes.

The lye and fats will not mix as they have different densities so don't be alarmed by the two layers that you see developing.

If you are mixing the mixture by hand, start stirring slowly to incorporate the two levels. If you are using a hand-held blender, put it into the mixture and tap a couple of times to release any air bubbles. Once it is completely covered, you can turn it on. Mixing by hand will take a lot longer, especially as the olive oil takes longer to trace. With the blender, this will take a couple of minutes.

You will know that the mixture is ready when it looks as though it is the same consistency as a milkshake that has melted a bit and is fully combined. Be careful not to over beat as then it will not be pourable.

Pour the mixture into your mould, being careful not to spill any onto yourself. If you find that the sides of the mould are bulging, shore it up by putting heavy books around the edges. The mould should be put in a place where it will be undisturbed for at least three days and you should cover it with card so that no dust can settle on the soap. Wrap in an old towel and leave it alone.

Check on the mixture after two-three days – it is ready to take out of the mould if the soap is cool and hard to the touch. If the soap is yielding or still warm, leave it in for longer.

You can now remove the mould and you should be able to cut your soap using a sharp, smooth blade. Set the bars up on your curing table or, if you don't have one, place a sheet of freezer paper on a shelf and stand them on that. Make sure that there is plenty of space for air to circulate around the bars and turn them every few days.

They will be completely ready for use after 6 weeks.

That is the basic process and you will follow a similar process for all soaps. Always melt semi-solid oils before incorporating them into the fat mixture and you'll be fine.

Calculating the Lye Content

Let's say that you've decided to use coconut oil. It has an SAP of 0.178. You then multiply the weight of the oil that you plan to use by the SAP to figure out how much lye you need. Let's say you've decided to use 5 ounces of coconut oil, for example, the calculation will be:

$5 \times 0.178 = 0.89$.

You will thus need around 0.89 ounces of lye to convert the oil to soap. If you want a more moisturizing soap, you can reduce the lye content by about 5% so that some of the oil is not saponified. I would not advise changing these numbers too much though – especially while you are learning.

Chapter 6: Natural Soap Cheat Sheet

Recipes Ready to Use Now

These are all made using the simple recipe in the previous chapter – the ingredients are added when the soap begins to trace. Alternatively, you can make the base plain and then re-batch it later with the following recipes.

Java Shower Soap

Add in 1.5 ounces of Benzoin essential oil and 1 tablespoon of coffee grounds for a soap that smells great and that will exfoliate and feed the skin at the same time. The coffee also gives the soap a nice color.

Soap for Sensitive Skin

This one requires that you change the basic recipe slightly by infusing the olive oil with dried calendula petals first. Use about an ounce of calendula petals. You can also add in about 0.5 ounces of dried calendula petals as a decorative feature for the soap. This soap is scented using 1.5 ounces of Sandalwood oil.

Honey and Oatmeal Soap

Add 0.4 ounces of honey and a cup of ground oatmeal to the soap. The oatmeal acts as an exfoliant and will also help soothe irritated skin. 1 ounce of Benzoin oil. The honey and the benzoin oil will moisturize the skin and give the soap a nice scent.

Lucky Lavender Soap

Add in an ounce of Lavender essential oil and some dried lavender leaves or petals. If you want to, add in purple coloring as well.

Citrus & Calendula Soap

Add 15ml of melted Shea butter to the re-batched soap while still warm and stir in well. Add in a handful of dried calendula petals and 0.5 ounces each of Grapefruit oil and Tangerine oil. Mix well and decant.

The above are just some ideas for the soaps that you can make. The range of soaps that you can make with the basic recipe is pretty much only limited by your imagination. Just keep to the basic volume rules when adding your fragrance oils and you should be fine.

Don't be afraid of mixing it up – once you have the basic recipe mastered, you can experiment away – some of my nicest batches of soaps have been a result of having come of experimenting.

Chapter 7:
Body Butter Basics

How To Make Your Own Body Butters

Making your own body butters is a lot simpler than making soaps and you do not have to use dangerous chemicals like lye. You will need to decide from the outset whether or not you will make your own base for the lotions from scratch or whether or not you will use a good quality organic base.

The Benefits of a Pre-Prepared Base

I am rather lucky in that we have a wonderful herbal store not far from us. They make a great organic base and you are able to buy it by the quart. I am perfectly happy using this base as I know the owners well and I trust them. I know that it is an organic base. They use a mixture of grape seed oil and sweet almond oil to make the base and I have been using it for years now. It is nice and thick and if I want to make it thicker, I warm it up and add in some Shea Butter.

It is far easier if you can source a base to use for your lotions instead of making them from scratch as emulsifying the fats can be tedious. That said, if you prefer to make them yourself, there is no problem with that and I will give you the recipe that I used before I started getting the pre-made base.

If, on the other hand, you can find a base that is organic and is from a trusted source, I don't feel that there is any problem in using that. All you really are doing is saving yourself some time and effort.

If you are making your own lotion from scratch, you will need oil such as olive oil, coconut oil, Shea butter, sweet almond oil or grape seed oils.

Coconut oil is not for everyone as it can be quite drying to the skin. There is also a possibility of the coconut oil causing a skin rash when used over time. It is a great cleanser and so could have a place as a part of your body butter - it should just not account for more than 20% of the total oils used. Coconut oil is semi-solid at room temperature so it should always be less than half the total mixture if you want the mixture to be more viscous in nature.

Lanolin is another fat that is often used in creams and lotions –Don't use it on the face because, although it is very moisturizing, it can promote hair growth. Lanolin is derived from sheep's wool so it is not suitable f you want to avoid animal products completely.

Sweet Almond oil is a good neutral choice for a cream because it can be used by people with all skin types. It is particularly good if you have dry or sensitive skin and it is well tolerated by those with oily skin as well. It is a good oil to use in a butter for treating stretch marks.

Grape Seed oil is better for people with normal to oily skin as it has a more astringent quality than sweet almond oil. It is a lighter base oil as well. What many therapists do is to mix it in equal quantities with sweet almond oil to create blends that are lighter in texture but just as nourishing.

Olive oil makes a good additive to the base of the cream - if using extra virgin olive oil, you can make up the base of the cream using olive oil - it is an excellent moisturizer, in some parts of Italy, women to this day use olive oil in place of other moisturizers. The reason that I suggest using extra virgin olive oil in your body butter is because it is not as heavily scented as the less refined grades of olive oil.

Shea butter is a very popular ingredient for lotions and creams because it is very moisturizing. It is solid at room temperature and feels harder than coconut oil so it should rather be used more as a special treatment oil than a main ingredient. Ordinarily it should not take up more than about 35% of the total oil content in your body butter. It will need to be melted before you can blend other oils in.

Emulsifying wax is something that you can source online and it is what will hold the lotion together in the end. If you don't want to use an emulsifying wax, you will need to create a water-in-oil emulsion rather than an oil-in-water emulsion. The major difference between the two is that the former tends to be a little greaser. It is easier to use the emulsifying wax and you will find that the body butters are better absorbed when you do.

Essential oils are the only thing that I use to scent my body butters and creams. They have a dual purpose because they also have healing properties in their own right. You don't need a lot – 1%-3% of the overall quantity is plenty. I have not listed all the essential oils here but I have listed my recipes for my favourite body butters and creams creams. There is tons of information online to help you choose what other essential oils will be suitable for you.

Botanical ingredients are very popular when it comes to body butters and lotions but you need to be very careful when adding them as they can make the cream go off faster. You can reduce the chances of the batch going off by adding a natural preservative like Vitamin E, by being very careful to sterilize the jars or by using infused oils or herbal teas as opposed to actual botanical matter. If you are using botanical ingredients, you also need to use distilled water as tap water could be hosting bacteria.

Colorants can be used if you really want to but I see no reason at all to color your body butters. If you do decide to color them, use cosmetic grade colorants. I believe that the more natural our beauty products are, the better they are for us. Ask yourself this question, "Does adding a colorant add any significant value?" If not, why bother adding it?

Vitamin E oil is a natural preservative that you can add to your creams. It also helps makes the creams more nourishing. Vitamin E can extend the shelf-life of your body butter quite extensively simply because it is such a potent anti-oxidant. You do not need to use a lot either - 5ml per batch of 500ml cream is sufficient.

Chapter 8:
Body Butter Cheat Sheet

Recipes Ready To Use Now

Your Base Recipe

1 part emulsifying wax

3 parts oil (I find adding equal quantities of sweet almond oil and grape seed oil makes a nice balanced lotion)

6 parts distilled water

Melt the oils and emulsifying wax in a double boiler on the stove. Heat the water separately. Check the temperatures of both mixes and when they are around about the same, slowly pour the water in whilst whisking the mixture well. Mix until the water and oils are properly incorporated and the mixture is creamy and thick.

Decant into sterilized containers and allow to cool.

The key here is to work slowly and steadily when adding the water to the mix. If you want to thicken the texture, you can allow the mix to cool and put it in the freezer for a about 20 minutes. Take out and whisk briskly. Repeat.

Adding In Extra Ingredients

Botanical Ingredients

If you are going to use botanical ingredients to your cream like fresh flower petals, warm the mixture in a double boiler and add in the petals. Bring to the boil and allow to simmer for 20 minutes. Once the twenty minutes are up, let strain the petals out.

The problem with using fresh ingredients here is that they can quite easily go off and cause your body butter to go bad. It is better to infuse the oils in this manner than to add in too many fresh ingredients to your creams.

Alternatively, if you do want to add fresh ingredients, make small batches at a time - batches that can be used in a week or so and store in the refrigerator.

Personally I feel that the fresh ingredient craze is a passing fad. I keep my fresh fruit to use on my skin as a treatment product rather than adding into the actual cream itself.

If your main aim in adding in fresh botanicals is to scent the body butter, you are better off using essential oils. The scent of the petals in the mixture added in this manner will be more herbal than floral because of the heat used to extract them.

Essential Oils

Add these in when the cream is cool and stir well with a wooden skewer/ stirring stick. Add the oils a drop at a time and re-evaluate the scents as you go along. This is time consuming at first but necessary to get the scent that you like. If you add too many drops of essential oils at a time, this is easily rectified by adding more of your base body butter.

Special Use Oils

Adding in special ingredients such as avocado oil or wheat germ oil, for example, can help rev up the lotion's potency.

These oils should be added when the lotion is cool and should account for no more than 5%-10% of the overall volume or they will have too much of an effect on the texture of the cream.

Vitamin E Oil

If using vitamin E oil as a preservative, add it in when the cream has been cooled. About 2% volume will be enough to help preserve your blend and will also boost the moisturizing power of your cream.

If you want to make a cream that is really a lot more effective, look at adding in a few of these ingredients:

Avocado oil is great for very dry or damaged skin. Keep it to a maximum of 10% volume as it is a very thick oil and can be sticky. It can also be useful when added to a treatment for dry hair. This oil does tend to have a shorter shelf-life so do only buy as much as you can use in 6 months or so.

Rose Hip oil is a wonderful skin regenerator and great for dry skin – I actually use it as it is as a serum before applying my night cream. You can add it to your lotion for extra oomph. It makes a wonderful addition to body butter, especially if you are wanting to get rid of scars or stretch marks.

Macadamia Nut oil is another skin soother and will extend the life of your blend. It is one of the oils with the longest life span and is particularly suited to dry and damaged skin and hair. It makes a good treatment for skin and hair that have had too much sun.

Olive oil can be added for extra moisturizing and dealing with troubled skin. In this case, you should use extra virgin olive oil. The oil has anti-bacterial properties and is deeply nourishing and can be used as your main oil in the body butter if you like.

Sandalwood and Cedar Wood Essential oils are a good choice to use as a fixative oil – both help to hydrate the skin and will help your oil maintain it scent longer.

Palmarosa Essential oil is one of the best oils to help regenerate skin and is one that I use often.

Geranium Essential oil is a balancing oil and helps to regenerate skin and is another that I use often. I don't like its scent – it is quite strong – so I will use about half the amount that I would for other oils but it is a good all-round remedy for treating irritated skin.

Castor oil is a popular ingredient in the beauty industry and is moisturizing and is used in a lot of soap recipes. Personally I feel that it is too sticky to use in a body butter – there are simply better options out there.

A Note on Perishable Ingredients

Perishable ingredients such as milk and cream should not be added to your mixture. They will go off very quickly and leave you with a lotion that looks and smells unpleasant.

It might sound like lots of fun to have a whipped cream body butter but, if you do add in real cream, you need to use the body butter within a few days of making it. If you do want to benefit by using dairy products, it is better to put them straight into you bathwater.

Recipes for Your Home Collection

Exotic Body Butter

450ml Basic lotion recipe

50ml Rose Hip oil

10 drops Sandalwood oil

10 drops Neroli oil

10 drops Palmarosa oil

10 drops Rose oil

Blend all the ingredients together and store in a sterilized jar. This body butter should only be applied at night because it has neroli oil in it and that can be photo-toxic. The sandalwood and rose hip oils in this mix make it particularly nourishing. The neroli, rose and palmarosa oil help to regenerate your skin. The overall scent of this cream is floral and pleasant. It also has a calming effect.

Special Night Serum

100 ml Rose Hip oil

5 drops Neroli oil

5 drops Rose oil

I know that this is not technically a body butter but I find that it is a wonderful treatment for dry skin. Apply just after your shower at night or after cleansing the skin and leave for about 5 minutes. Blot excess with a tissue.

Daybreak Butter

500ml Basic lotion recipe

5 drops Geranium oil

10 drops Lavender oil

10 drops Palmarosa oil

10 drops Sandalwood oil

Blend all the ingredients well and store in a sterilized jar. There are no special use oils in this blend because the cream that you use during the day should be lighter in texture. If you feel that your skin needs extra help, replace 50ml of the basic cream recipe for one of the special use oils. The lavender and geranium oils promote regeneration and balance the skin.

Body Bliss Butter

450 ml Basic lotion recipe

50ml Extra virgin olive oil

50ml Sweet almond oil

10 drops Ylang Ylang oil

10 drops Neroli oil

10 drops Sandalwood oil

10 drops Rose oil

10 drops Jasmine oil

Blend all the oils together and store in a sterilized jar. The ylang ylang and jasmine lend an exotic scent to the oil and the others help with regenerating the skin. There are a lot of different oils in this recipe but they blend together really well for a heavenly scent.

Skin Cleansing Cream

450ml Basic lotion recipe

50ml Sweet almond oil – if your skin is dry OR

50ml Grape seed oil – if your skin is oilier

10 Drops Neroli oil

10 Drops Sandalwood oil

 Use this as a cream cleanser in winter if your skin is dry or mature.

Eczema Soothing Body Butter - Suitable for Baby's Bum Too!

500ml Basic lotion recipe

10 drops Geranium oil

10 drops Palmarosa oil

10 drops Sandalwood oil

When nothing else worked for my eczema, this cream really was a winner. I also made a batch form my sister-in-law to use as a baby bum cream on my niece and nephew and it really helped. The smell of the cream is a little herbal but it is worth using it for the results.

Acne Treatment/ Butter

450ml Basic lotion recipe (use grape seed oil as your primary oil here)

15 Drops Geranium oil

10 Drops Lavender oil

10 Drops Palmarosa oil

10 drops Cedar Wood oil

If you have acne anywhere on your body, it is important to be gentler with your skin or you will inflame it even more. Cleanse only twice a day, no more and apply this butter every night. I know that a lot has been said about Tea Tree oil but I am not keen on its scent so I don't actually use it often. I find that this recipe works a lot better than Tea Tree oil as it is not as harsh.

Super Relaxing Body Butter

125ml Magnesium flakes dissolved in 45ml boiled water

67.5ml Coconut oil

30ml Emulsifying wax or beeswax

45ml Shea butter

Set aside the magnesium mixture to cool. Using a double boiler, combine the rest of the ingredients and set your burner to medium. Once these have combined completely, remove from the heat and leave to cool. When it reaches room temperature, transfer it to a long jar and, using your hand-held blender set to medium, blend together. At the same time, add in the magnesium mixture very slowly. Continue blending until everything is mixed together and refrigerate for 20 minutes. Blend again to get the right consistency.

The magnesium in this mixture will help to soften the skin and help to ease aching muscles. It also provides a little protection from the sun.

Honey Bun Body Butter

60ml Coconut oil

30ml Beeswax

17.5ml Extra virgin olive oil

5ml Honey

30ml Lanolin

45ml Aloe Vera gel

5 Drops Sandalwood oil

5 drops Lavender oil

1 Vitamin E caplet

Place the first 4 ingredients into a double boiler. Set your burner to Medium-High and allow to melt. Repeat this process with a second double burner, this time using only the aloe gel. When they are around about the same temperature, mix together. Mix in the lanolin and then reduce the heat to low. Stir in the remaining ingredients and whisk until smooth and creamy.

Deliciously Divine Body Butter

45 g Cocoa butter

45 g Macadamia nut oil

90 g Shea butter

10 Drops Rosemary oil

20 Drops Peppermint oil

Measure out all your ingredients first. Place the cocoa butter in a heat-proof mixing bowl and add the Shea butter and macadamia nut oil next. Place in a double boiler, set you burner to medium and heat until the oils are melted. Remove from the heat and allow to cool for around 10 minutes. Place in the freezer for around 20 minutes. Beat with an electric beater for 5 minutes on high and then put back into the freezer for another 20 minutes. Beat for another 5 minutes until it turns creamy. Now that the mixture is cold, you can add in the essential oils – beat one last time. Refrigerate between uses.

Easy Body Butter

7 oz. Shea Butter

500ml Coconut oil

1 drop Tea Tree Oil

20 drops of the essential oil of your choice

Put the Shea butter and coconut oil into a double boiler. Set your burner to medium and heat until completely combined. Stir if necessary. Remove from the heat and allow to cool for around 10 minutes. Place in the freezer for around 20 minutes. Beat with an electric beater for 5 minutes on high and then put back into the freezer for another 20 minutes. Beat for another 5 minutes until it turns creamy. Now that the mixture is cold, you can add in the essential oils – beat one last time. Refrigerate between uses.

Extra Moisturizing Body Butter

250ml Shea butter

125ml Beef tallow

125ml Jojoba oil

5ml Peppermint oil

10ml Vitamin E oil

Put the tallow and Shea butter in a double boiler and heat until completely melted. Take off the heat and mix in the Jojoba oil. Allow to cool for about half an hour and then stir in the rest of the ingredients.

Place in the freezer for 20 minutes. Whip thoroughly using an electric mixer and repeat until desired consistency is achieved.

Tropical Heat Body Butter

25g Cocoa butter

10g Jojoba or Beeswax wax

25 g Mango butter

30g Shea butter

5ml Sweet Almond oil

5ml Vitamin E oil

5 Drops Sweet Orange oil

5 Drops Lemon oil

10 Drops Lime oil

Place the first 4 ingredients in a double boiler. Set your burner to low and leave for 20 minutes. Mix in the Sweet Almond oil and the Vitamin E oil and mix well. If necessary, leave the mixture on the heat until it is completely melted.

Allow to cool slightly before adding in the essential oils. Whisk to the desired consistency.

Vanilla Benzoin Butter

125ml Sweet almond oil

250ml Cocoa butter

125ml Coconut oil

1 Vanilla bean

Place butter and coconut oil in a double boiler and set your burner to medium. When melted, remove from the heat and leave for half an hour. Grind the vanilla up fine and stir in with the Sweet Almond oil and the coconut oil mix. Put in the the freezer for about 20 minutes. Use an electric mixer to beat. Repeat until required consistency is achieved.

Lemon Whip Body Butter

90ml Coconut oil

67.5ml Cacao butter

5ml Vitamin E oil

4 Drops Lemon oil

Put the coconut oil and Shea butter in a double boiler and heat until completely melted. Take off the heat. Allow to cool for about half an hour and then stir in the rest of the ingredients.

Place in the freezer for 20 minutes. Whip thoroughly using an electric mixer and repeat until desired consistency is achieved.

Yummy Chocolate Body Butter

125ml Cocoa butter

125ml Shea butter

125ml Coconut oil

125ml Jojoba oil

20 Drops Peppermint oil

30ml Cacao powder

30ml Vitamin E oil

Put the cocoa butter and Shea butter in a double boiler and set your burner to medium. Heat until completely melted. Stir in the coconut oil and allow to melt. Take off the heat.

In a separate bowl, slowly mix the cocoa powder and the Jojoba oil. Mix until smooth and then add to the warm mixture. Allow to cool for about half an hour and then stir in the rest of the ingredients.

Place in the freezer for 20 minutes. Whip thoroughly using an electric mixer and repeat until desired consistency is achieved.

Golden Honey Butter

1.4 oz Shea butter

0.4 oz Cocoa butter

1 oz Extra virgin olive oil

0.5 oz Beeswax

1.5 oz Coconut oil

0.7 oz Raw, organic honey

2.5ml Borax

5 oz distilled water

10 Drops Neroli oil

5 Drops Jasmine oil

5 Drops Ylang Ylang oil

Mix the Borax into the distilled water and set aside. Put all the ingredients aside from the essential oils into a double boiler and set your burner to medium. Heat until completely melted. Take off the heat and stir in the borax solution. Blend well using you hand-held blender.

Allow to cool for about half an hour and then stir in the essential oils.

Place in the freezer for 20 minutes. Whip thoroughly using an electric mixer and repeat until desired consistency is achieved.

Irritation Free Body Butter

250ml Shea Butter

125ml Coconut oil

125ml Sweet Almond oil

22.5ml Beeswax

15ml Zinc Oxide

15ml Glycerin

10 Drops Lavender oil

10 Drops Chamomile oil

Put the coconut oil, beeswax, Sweet Almond oil and Shea butter in a double boiler and heat until completely melted. Take off the heat. Add in the Zinc Oxide and the Glycerin. Allow to cool for about half an hour and then stir in the essential oils.

Place in the freezer for 20 minutes. Whip thoroughly using an electric mixer and repeat until desired consistency is achieved.

Chapter 9:
Shampoo Heaven

The Basics of Creating Your Own Shampoo

We all know that we should eat well and avoid over-styling our hair to keep it in tip-top shape. That is something that we know but it is not always something that we follow through on.

Fortunately, essential oils can go a long way to helping nourish the hair and conditioning the scalp. Rosemary oil, West Indian Bay oil and Clary Sage oil are all great t0 help bring an oily scalp back into balance and kill off any bacteria. Use diluted in oil and rub into the scalp. Rosemary can stimulate new hair growth and help to condition hair. Used in a rinse, it can help to maintain the color of dark hair. Use Chamomile oils in a rinse for light hair to help it shine.

Lavender oil helps to untangle hair when used in the rinse water and, when rubbed into the scalp, helps to condition it.

You can add a couple of drops of Lavender or Rosemary oils to your shampoo or conditioner to easily incorporate them into your hair care routine. Alternatively you can make your own shampoo by grating a bar of castile soap into a cup of warm water and allowing it to dissolve in there.

Oil treatments are the best conditioners for hair - even if you have greasy hair, you should use an oil treatment once a week. In most cases, you will warm up the oil a little, add your chosen essential oils and then rub the oil into the scalp - If you have greasy hair, stop here. If your hair is dry or frazzled, massage the mixture through to the end of the hair shaft. Wrap your hair and scalp in cling film and a warm towel to really intensify the treatment and leave on for at least 20 minutes.

When you are ready to wash the oil out of the hair, you do not wash your hair as normal. Instead of wetting your hair first and then applying the shampoo, you will mix the shampoo into a handful of water and then massage that into the scalp and ends of the hair. Rinse and repeat and the oil should be gone.

Always remember that you do need to change your treatments up once in a while to prevent your hair from developing a tolerance for the shampoos that you make.

Use the clarifying treatments once or twice a week to reduce residue left by styling products.

Amla Oil

If you can get hold of Amla oil, also known as Indian Gooseberry oil, you can use it as carrier oil for your other oils. The trick with Amla oil is to only rub it into your scalp - do not massage into the shaft of the hair itself as this can leave the hair feeling dry. Rub into the scalp and leave on overnight. When you rinse it off the next morning, you will be amazed at how soft and manageable your hair becomes.

Warming Oil for Hair Treatments

All you need to do is to measure out the oil that you are going to use and put it into a wide-mouthed jar. Boil the kettle and find a bowl that the jar fits into and stand the jar in it. When the kettle has boiled, pour boiling water into the bowl so that it surrounds the jar of oil and reaches about half-way up the jar. Let the oil stand for about 10 minutes to warm nicely.

Alternatively you can warm the oil in the microwave but do be careful doing this or you could make it too hot. Warm for a minute on a lower setting - you want the oil to be at skin temperature when you use it, not scalding.

Chapter 10:
Shampoo Cheat Sheet

Recipes Ready To Use Now

The Ultimate Hair Conditioner for Oily Hair

This helps to condition the hair and to stimulate growth.

25ml Olive oil, slightly warmed.

5 Drops Rosemary oil

5 Drops Lavender oil

Warm the oil using the method mentioned above. Add the oils. Apply to the scalp, massaging in. Wrap your head in cling wrap and a warm towel. Leave on for 20 minutes before rinsing out.

The Ultimate Hair Conditioner for Dry Hair

25ml Jojoba oil, slightly warmed

5 Drops Vertiver oil

5 Drops Lavender oil

Warm the oil using the method mentioned above. Add the oils. Apply to the scalp, massaging in. Wrap your head in cling wrap and a warm towel. Leave on for 20 minutes before rinsing out.

On the Go Scalp Rub

5 Drops Lavender oil

5 Drops Tea Tree oil

Massage the oils into your scalp and carry on with your day. You do not need to rinse them out of your hair.

Hair Tonic

10 Drops Rosemary/ Chamomile oils (Depending on whether your hair is dry or not)

1 Tablespoon of Apple Cider Vinegar

100ml Lavender or Rose Water

Mix the ingredients together well and then massage into the scalp. Leave on for at least half an hour or overnight. If you can get away with it, do not rinse out until the next time you need to wash your hair, the longer it stays on, the better.

Dry Shampoo

1 Drop Rosemary oil

1 Tablespoon Fuller's Earth or Powdered Orris Root

Mix the powder and the Rosemary oil together and apply to the greasy parts of your head. Leave in place for about 5 minutes so that excess oil can be absorbed.

Dry Brittle Hair Treatment

125ml Mayonnaise

A few drops of shampoo

Tepid water

5 Drops Lavender essential oil

5 Drops Sandalwood essential oil

Mix mayo with shampoo add enough lukewarm water to make a paste. Mix in the oils and apply to hair after a regular shampoo. Leave on 10 minutes and then shampoo out.

Homemade Scented Hair Gel

250ml Water

30ml Flax seed

2 Drops essential oils of your choice

Soak the seeds in the water overnight. The next day, bring to the boil on the stove, adding more water if necessary. As soon as the mixture boils, remove from the heat. Leave for about half an hour to cool and set. Strain through a sieve or muslin. Leave to cool completely and then mix in your oils. Use as you would a commercial gel.

Hot Oil Hair Treatment

30ml olive oil

15ml honey

2 Drops Lavender essential oil

Mix honey and olive oil in a small plastic bag and seal. Fill a coffee cup with water that has just stopped short of boiling and put bag into it to allow oils to heat up. Remove from water and add the Lavender oil. Massage into your hair from scalp through to the tips. Put a shower cap on and then cover your hair with a towel to boost the treatment. Leave for at least 20 minutes before shampooing out.

Revitalizing Avocado Hair Treatment

1 Avocado -- peeled and pitted

30ml Honey

5 drops Lavender oil

5 Drops Chamomile oil

Mash the avocado and mix in the other ingredients. Apply to the hair an leave in for half an hour before shampooing out.

Chamomile Shampoo

4 Bags of Chamomile tea

5 Drops Chamomile oil

375ml Water, just boiled

60ml pure soap flakes

22.5ml Glycerin

Let the tea bags steep in the water for 10 minutes. Remove the bags and add the soap flakes. Let stand until the soap softens. Stir in glycerin and essential oils until mixture is well blended. Use as normal.

Dry Shampoo

125ml Cornstarch

5 Drops of the essential oil of your choice.

Mix together the oil and the cornstarch and sprinkle over greasy hair. Rub it in gently and leave for a couple of minutes. Brush out again for clean-looking, oil-free hair.

Sprinkle the cornstarch in your hair, let it absorb for a few minutes, brush it out. This is great if you are in a pinch.

Deep Conditioner

1 Small jar of real mayonnaise

1/2 An avocado, peeled and pitted

5 ml Sandalwood oil

5ml Lavender oil

5 ml Neroli oil

Mix everything together well and the massage into scalp and all along the hair shafts. Put on a shower cap and then put a warm towel over this and leave in place for half an hour before shampooing out.

Rosemary Conditioner

10 Drops Rosemary essential oil

5 Drops Lavender essential oil

150ml Sweet Almond oil

Mix well together and apply to scalp and ends of the hair. Wrap with a shower cap and warm towel and leave on for half an hour before rinsing out. (This is a very stimulating treatment so it is best reserved for use in the morning or early afternoon.)

Egg Conditioner Recipe

5ml Sweet Almond oil

2 drops Chamomile oil

1 egg yolk

1 cup water

Beat the egg yolk until it is frothy, add the oil then beat again. Add to the water. Massage into the scalp and throughout your hair. Rinse well.

Oily Hair Treatment

2.5ml Aloe Vera gel

5ml Lemon juice

1 Drop Rosemary oil

Blend ingredients together with 1/4 cup of your regular hair shampoo. Wash hair then rinse well.

Hair Product Buildup Remover

75ml Apple Cider vinegar

250ml Water

10 Drops Juniper Berry oil

After conditioning the hair use this as a final rinse. Leaves your hair soft and shiny.

Clean as a Whistle Shampoo

187.5ml Distilled water

125ml Natural shampoo

2.5ml Fine table salt

5 ml Witch hazel

5ml Sweet almond oil

7 Drops Jasmine oil

3 Drops Ylang-Ylang oil

Dissolve the salt in the water and then add to witch hazel. Mix in the shampoo and the oils and blend well. Massage into hair, leave to soak for about two minutes and then rinse out again.

Chapter 11:

Packaging and Storing Your Creations

Your Guide to Keeping Your New Products in Tip Top Shape

Now that you have taken the time to make your own soaps, shampoos and body butters, it is important to think a little bit about how to best preserve their efficacy. These are not like store-bought products that have an indefinite shelf-life and the essential oils can lose their potency over time. In this chapter we go through packaging and storing your products for best results and also some ideas on how to package them if you are giving them as gifts.

Natural Soaps

What amazes most people about home-made soap is how well it keeps its color and fragrance without the need for preservatives. Soap, when stored properly, can last for years. In fact, pure castile soap has been known to last an amazing 20 years without going off at all.

The shelf-life of the soap will depend on the ingredients in it. You can add a fresh fruit or vegetable puree if you like but this will decrease the shelf-life of your soap to less than a year. You also risk mould growing on the soaps while they are curing so it is best to avoid fresh ingredients.

The simpler the recipe, the more likely the soap will last for longer.

That said, if you are making soaps for yourself, make enough to last about a year at a time or less. You can always make more later if you need to.

The scent is where you may find problems occurring – some scents, such as the more volatile citrus essential oils will dissipate more quickly over time so this should be kept in mind.

When packaging cold-process soaps, you have a lot of options – the soaps do not have to be packed in cling-film to keep them free of moisture build-up so you can choose a much wider range of packaging options than you can with melt and pour soaps.

Natural soaps can even be left unwrapped if you like although this will allow the scent to dissipate faster. What I normally do is to wrap the soaps for my own personal use in plain brown paper bags. That way, after the soap is finished, the wrapper is nicely scented and I can use it as a drawer liner.

Here are some ideas that you can use if you want to make a gift of the soaps:

Soap Block or Dish

You can simply find a nice soap block or dish to match your soap. If using a block, a more rustic look can be achieved by tying it to the dish using plain raffia. If you like, add a couple of sticks of cinnamon before tying on the raffia.

If you have found a pretty soap dish, you can play with a more feminine packaging. Tie to the dish using ribbon or lace trim. If you like, add a dried flower before tying to make it look prettier.

Button It Up

A plainer soap can be wrapped in newspaper or brown paper for something a little more different. Tie the parcel with string and thread a pretty button through before tying your bow.

Scrap Happy

Choose a lovely piece of scrap-booking paper to cover your soap in. You can then affix a label to the front or wrap with a band of co-ordinating paper to finish it off.

A Soapy Bucket

Look at the dollar store for those small, metal mini-buckets to place your bar of soap in. Wrap the soap in tissue paper, half-fill the bucket with straw/ tissue paper and then set your soap in it. You can further decorate the bucket using a pretty bow or pretty it up using raffia.

A Candy Gift

Look out at candy-making supply stores for boxes with clear windows to display the soap. You can even find fun moulds that make the soap look like candy. It is important then to clearly label the boxes so people know that the "candy" is not edible.

Colorful Cellophane

Cellophane can make for a great packaging material when you need a pop of color or some extra oomph. Cut it into strips to use as a base packing material to set off colourful soaps or use it to wrap your soaps directly.

Lovely in Lace

If you really want to pretty up your cold-process soap, look for a lovely piece of lace to wrap it in. Finish it off with a matching ribbon.

Vintage Labels

There are plenty of free printable vintage soap wrappers that you can find online or you can design your own at a site like Canva.com. If you are planning to sell the soap, however, you must make sure that you can use these commercially before printing them out.

All that is really required for a great vintage label is some off-white printing paper. Wrap your soap in a layer of wax wrap and then wrap with the vintage soap wrapper to finish it off.

Sweet And Simple

Tissue paper can be a great to make soaps look really pretty. Again, wrap in a layer of wax wrap before wrapping with the tissue paper. Finish off with a matching trim or ribbon.

Body Butters

I love those short little mason jars when it comes to giving the body butters as gifts. That, with a nice little label is all that is really needed.

As with all essential oil products, it is better if you use glass to store them in. Choose containers that are easy to decant the butter into and containers that make it easy to get the butter out of - it is not as viscous as a lotion is so this could be a problem.

Shampoos

A bottle that seals well is the best bet here. Again, glass is the better option but you can use plastic as well if you really want to.

Olive oil bottles are quite nice to use as an alternative container, as long as they are properly cleaned and rinsed out.

Conclusion

Thank you again for downloading this book!

I do hope that this has been a thorough introduction into the world of making your own natural soaps, body butters and shampoos.

All you now need to do is to try out the recipes and let the results speak for themselves. Making your own beauty products is fun and creative and, best of all, at the end of the day you have something that is completely unique, that smells great and that is really effective. You'll wonder how you ever managed before without making your own products.

I would like to ask you one favor, if you don't mind. Would you please rate this book on Amazon for me? It is really important for a self-publisher like me and I would really appreciate it. Thank you so much!

Good luck with your future crafting!

www.ingramcontent.com/pod-product-compliance
Lightning Source LLC
Chambersburg PA
CBHW071215280526
45787CB00002B/699